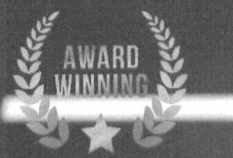

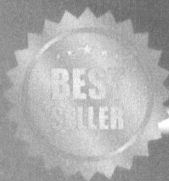

THE PROCESSED PANTRY

Our Love Affair with Engineered Eats

I0437658

R. ORBIT

Disclaimer:

This book is intended as a general guide to the topic of processed foods and their influence on our food habits. While every effort has been made to ensure that the information contained within is accurate and up-to-date, it is not intended as a substitute for professional advice or treatment. Readers are encouraged to consult with a healthcare provider for nutritional guidance and support.

978-1-4467-7996-5
Imprint: Lulu.com

In "The Processed Pantry: Our Love Affair with Engineered Eats", Robbie Orbit explores our complicated relationship with processed foods. Dive into the world of flavor engineering, the chemistry of additives, and the socio-economic impacts of these readily available, easy-to-consume products. Orbit unravels why these foods are designed to be irresistible, and how they've shaped our global food patterns, health, and society. A compelling and illuminating read for anyone interested in understanding our modern food landscape.

This book is dedicated to all those seeking clarity in the convoluted world of food choices we face today. May you find the strength to navigate towards healthier and more sustainable paths.

FORWARD

It's easy to demonize processed foods. We see them lined up on supermarket shelves, often gaudily packaged, teeming with ingredients we can't pronounce, and we are regularly reminded of their potential detriments to our health. But processed foods, for better or worse, are an indelible part of our modern lives, offering convenience, affordability, and a certain level of predictability in an ever-changing world.

Robbie Orbit's "The Processed Pantry: Our Love Affair with Engineered Eats" is a comprehensive exploration into the intricate world of processed foods. This book is not a sweeping condemnation, but rather a considered study of these foods, exploring why we are drawn to them, and their impact on our health, society, and the planet.

What struck me most about this book is its balanced approach. Yes, there are chapters detailing the less savory aspects of processed foods - the high levels of sugars, salts, unhealthy fats, the role they play in global health crises such as obesity and heart disease, the environmental footprint. Yet, there is also an examination of how processed foods have shaped our lives, catering to our increasingly busy schedules, providing longer shelf lives, and making certain nutrients more readily available.

More importantly, Orbit challenges us, the readers, to critically engage with the choices we make at the dinner table. This book delves deep into the strategies we can adopt to strike a balance in our diets, to make informed decisions that promote our health, without entirely giving up on the convenience that processed foods offer.

"The Processed Pantry: Our Love Affair with Engineered Eats" also offers a glimpse into a future where processed foods can be part of the solution, not just the problem. It explores how technological innovation and shifting consumer preferences can pave the way for a new generation of processed foods that offer both nutrition and convenience.

Whether you're an avid foodie, a health-conscious consumer, a policy maker, or just someone interested in understanding more about the food you consume, this book is an enlightening read. It nudges us to look beyond the labels, to make better food choices, and to realize our collective power in shaping a healthier, more sustainable food future.

As you embark on this journey with Robbie Orbit, I encourage you to approach it with an open mind. This isn't just a book about processed foods; it's a book about us - our tastes, our habits, our choices, and our future. So, let's take a moment to examine our own pantry, to understand our relationship with processed foods, and to start a conversation that extends beyond ourselves, towards a healthier, more sustainable world.

Jada Nista

The Processed Pantry

As we walk down the grocery store aisle, rows upon rows of brightly packaged goods greet us, their alluring labels promising everything from low-calorie indulgence to hearty nourishment. These processed foods have woven themselves intricately into the fabric of our daily lives. But what exactly constitutes processed food?

The term "processed food" refers to any food item that has undergone a series of operations such as cooking, canning, freezing, dehydration, or milling to transform raw ingredients into a form that is more convenient, digestible, and palatable for the consumer. Processed foods range from the benign, such as washed and bagged spinach or roasted coffee beans, to the more vilified "ultra-processed" foods, including sugary breakfast cereals, fast food burgers, and microwaveable meals.

The era of processed foods dawned with the advent of industrialization in the 19th century. As societies became more urbanized, the demand for preserved, easily transportable foods grew. The invention of Nicolas Appert's canning technique in 1809 came as a groundbreaking solution, paving the way for food processing on a mass scale. Since then, the food processing industry has developed in leaps and bounds, paralleling technological advancement.

Many processed foods have shaped history in remarkable ways. Take, for example, condensed milk, a product born out of necessity during the American Civil War. The Union Army required a reliable source of milk that wouldn't spoil on the battlefield, and Gail Borden's condensed milk fit the bill. Post-war, it transitioned from a survival staple to a beloved ingredient, making its way into kitchens and sweet treats across the country.

However, it's important to distinguish between different levels of processing. Not all processed foods are detrimental to health. Pasteurized milk, frozen fruits and vegetables, and canned legumes are examples of minimally processed foods that retain much of their nutritional integrity. These products, often termed "convenience foods," have contributed significantly to the democratization of nutritious food, enabling individuals with limited time, cooking skills, or resources to access a more varied diet.

As we delve further into the higher tiers of processing, the picture becomes more complex. Foods processed to the point where they bear little resemblance to their original form, often laden with added sugars, fats, and salts, as well as a cocktail of food additives, dominate this category. These are the ultra-processed foods that have raised numerous public health concerns.

In essence, processed foods have been both a boon and a bane. They have revolutionized the way we eat, enabling longer shelf life, preserving the safety of food, and providing year-round availability of seasonal produce. However, in this transformation, we've also invited a host of health issues linked to overconsumption of ultra-processed products.

To truly understand our relationship with processed foods, we need to examine the myriad factors that play into their creation, consumption, and consequences. From flavor engineering to the psychology of food marketing, from socio-economic considerations to the global health implications - each facet provides a critical piece of the puzzle.

The world of processed foods is as intricate and multi-layered as the foods themselves. Through the subsequent chapters, we'll embark on a journey of exploration into this fascinating landscape, illuminating the role of processed foods in shaping our tastes, habits, and health.

T he roots of food processing are as old as human civilization itself. The story of processed foods is not a modern tale spun by industrialization, but a chronicle dating back to our earliest ancestors. It's a narrative of survival, innovation, and human ingenuity, deeply entwined with the history of civilization and the progress of technology.

Around 2 million years ago, our ancestors, the Homo habilis, discovered the power of processing food by using tools to pound and crush tough tubers and nuts, making these foods easier to eat and digest. This early form of food processing heralded a significant evolutionary milestone, enabling the growth of our brains and the development of our species.

Fire, discovered about 1.5 million years ago, revolutionized food processing. Cooking not only made food safer to eat by eliminating pathogens, but it also made it more digestible and palatable. Our Homo erectus ancestors who mastered fire and cooking had the competitive edge, gaining more energy from less food and boosting their survival.

Fast forward to around 10,000 B.C., with the dawn of agriculture in the Neolithic Revolution, food preservation became vital. The onset of crop cultivation and animal husbandry brought about seasonal food surpluses. To prevent this bounty from spoiling, early methods like sun-drying, smoking, fermenting, and salting were developed. These rudimentary forms of food processing allowed our ancestors to survive harsh winters and food shortages, facilitating the shift from nomadic to settled societies.

As civilizations flourished, so did the art of food processing. The Egyptians, around 3,500 B.C., were adept at milling wheat into flour to make bread, and they used salt to cure fish and meat. In ancient Rome, winemaking and olive oil production became sophisticated industries.

The exploration and colonization era of the 15th to 17th centuries spurred the need for long-lasting, transportable food. Salt-cured meat, hardtack biscuits, and pickled vegetables became staples on voyages. However, these preservation methods often fell short in nutritional adequacy, leading to conditions like scurvy among seafarers.

A significant breakthrough in food processing came in the early 19th century with Nicolas Appert's invention of canning. A French confectioner, Appert devised a method to preserve food by heating it in glass jars sealed with wax and reinforced with wire. By 1810, Englishman Peter Durand had patented the use of tin-coated iron cans instead of glass, laying the foundation of the modern canned food industry.

The late 19th and early 20th centuries saw the burgeoning of the industrial revolution, and with it, a seismic shift in food processing. The era's scientific and technological innovations, such as pasteurization, mechanical refrigeration, and assembly line production, made food processing more efficient, safe, and scalable. New processed products like breakfast cereals, canned pineapple, condensed milk, and carbonated beverages became popular.

In the mid-20th century, the fast-paced post-war era ushered in convenience foods: frozen dinners, instant noodles, TV dinners, and more. Processed foods morphed from a necessity into a lifestyle choice, epitomizing modernity, convenience, and affluence.

In the late 20th and early 21st centuries, the rise of global food corporations, advancements in food science and technology, and changes in dietary patterns fueled the ubiquity of ultra-processed foods. These foods, characterized by their long ingredient lists and high levels of sugar, fat, and salt, have become a dietary mainstay in many parts of the world, despite growing health concerns.

The history of processed foods is a mirror reflecting human progress, technological triumphs, and societal transformations. However, it also throws into sharp relief the profound challenges we face today: rampant chronic diseases, nutritional inequalities, and environmental issues. As we navigate these complexities, understanding the historical context of processed foods can shed light on potential pathways towards healthier, more sustainable food systems.

From pre-packaged salads to microwaveable dinners, our food landscape is brimming with products designed for our convenience. These ready-to-eat or ready-to-heat products have become a dietary staple, saving time in an era when many people are time-poor but task-rich. In understanding our relationship with processed foods, it's essential to grasp the crucial role that convenience plays in our food choices.

The concept of convenience in food extends far beyond mere preparation time. It encompasses various elements such as accessibility, portability, longer shelf-life, and easy storage. Convenience foods liberate us from the time-consuming tasks of meal planning, shopping for individual ingredients, food preparation, and cleaning up.

In the 1950s and 60s, as more women joined the workforce, the demand for convenience foods grew exponentially. Households with dual-income earners had less time for cooking, making processed foods an attractive option. Today, with the rise in single-person households, extended work hours, and the intensification of the "time squeeze," convenience foods have become a cornerstone of the modern diet.

Accessibility and portability further underscore the convenience of processed foods. Snack foods like granola bars, potato chips, or packaged sandwiches are easy to transport and consume on the go. For people with busy schedules, these foods cater to the need for mobile meals that fit into their active lifestyles.

Moreover, convenience foods provide a degree of predictability and control. Regardless of where you are in the world, a fast-food burger or a soda tastes virtually the same. This consistency can be comforting in unfamiliar situations and minimizes the risk of an "unpalatable" experience.

The longer shelf life of processed foods is another convenience aspect. Thanks to techniques like canning, freezing, and the use of preservatives, these foods can be stored for months or even years without spoiling. This durability not only reduces the frequency of grocery shopping but also provides a reliable food source in emergency situations or when fresh foods are unavailable.

While convenience foods offer numerous benefits, it's also necessary to consider their nutritional cost. Many of these foods are high in added sugars, fats, and sodium, and low in fiber and essential nutrients, contributing to a host of health issues such as obesity, diabetes, heart disease, and certain types of cancer. Furthermore, excessive reliance on convenience foods can lead to reduced cooking skills and a disconnection from our food's origins and the cultural practices surrounding meal preparation and communal dining.

In conclusion, convenience is a major driving force behind our reliance on processed foods. As our lives become busier, the allure of quick, easy meals grows stronger. Balancing this need for convenience with healthful choices is one of the key challenges in our contemporary food environment. It's a complex issue, necessitating a multifaceted approach that includes improving the nutritional quality of processed foods, educating consumers about healthy eating, and addressing broader societal factors that influence our food choices.

What makes a steaming bowl of macaroni and cheese so comforting, or the crunch of potato chips so satisfying? The answers lie within the fascinating science of taste, a complex sensory system that plays a fundamental role in our food preferences and dietary behaviors.

Taste perception begins with our taste buds, specialized sensory receptors embedded within the papillae on our tongues. Each taste bud is a bundle of 50 to 150 gustatory cells that respond to five basic tastes: sweet, salty, sour, bitter, and umami. When we eat, food molecules stimulate these cells, sending signals to our brain, which decodes these messages into taste sensations.

Sweetness, provided by sugars and certain other compounds, is universally liked and signals the presence of energy-rich carbohydrates in food. The love for sweetness is hardwired in us from birth; even newborns have been shown to prefer sweet tastes.

Salty taste, primarily triggered by sodium, enhances the flavors of many foods and is crucial in maintaining our body's fluid balance. However, our preference for salt is believed to be learned rather than innate, driven by dietary exposure.

Sourness is the taste that corresponds to the basic taste sensation of acidity. While mildly sour foods like citrus fruits are often considered refreshing, extreme sourness, as a natural warning sign of spoiled or unripe food, can be unpleasant.

Bitterness, triggered by a wide variety of compounds, acts as a natural warning system for potential toxins, as many poisonous substances taste bitter. Although we are biologically predisposed to reject bitter foods, repeated exposure can lead to acceptance and even preference for some bitter foods like coffee, dark chocolate, and leafy greens.

Umami, the fifth basic taste, was identified by Japanese scientist Kikunae Ikeda in 1908. It's described as a savory or meaty taste, imparted by foods high in the amino acid glutamate, like tomatoes, mushrooms, cheese, and meat.

The food industry strategically leverages these taste characteristics to engineer products that deliver an optimal taste experience. Sweetness and saltiness, in particular, are used extensively in processed foods to enhance palatability. The notorious "bliss point," a term coined by food scientist Howard Moskowitz, refers to the precise concentration of sweetness or saltiness that makes a food most enjoyable.

Beyond the five basic tastes, our eating experience is also profoundly influenced by other sensory attributes such as aroma, texture, temperature, color, and even sound. This multi-sensory integration contributes to what scientists call "flavor," a more holistic perception of our food.

Notably, our taste preferences aren't merely a matter of biology. They are shaped by a host of factors, including cultural practices, dietary habits, psychological influences, and even our genetic makeup. Certain genes can affect the density of taste buds on our tongues or our sensitivity to specific tastes, making us "supertasters," "tasters," or "non-tasters."

As we unravel the science of taste, we gain valuable insights into why we like the foods we do and why processed foods, engineered to tantalize our taste buds, often prove irresistible. In the next chapter, we delve deeper into how the food industry employs this science to create hyper-palatable products that keep us coming back for more.

F rom the perfectly salted crunch of a potato chip to the sweet burst of a gummy bear, processed foods can deliver taste experiences that are nothing short of addictive. Behind these flavors is an intricate science and art known as flavor engineering, which the food industry leverages to create products that not only taste good but are irresistibly craveable.

Flavor engineering encompasses the strategic manipulation of taste, aroma, texture, and appearance to optimize food palatability. Central to this process is an understanding of our sensory system's response to these different attributes and our physiological and psychological reactions to them. The aim is to hit the 'bliss point,' the exact level at which consumers derive the most pleasure from a product.

Taste manipulation is the cornerstone of flavor engineering. Processed foods are often loaded with sugar, salt, and fat - all of which are universally loved and stimulate our brains' reward system, driving us to seek out these foods repeatedly. The savory taste of umami, often enhanced through monosodium glutamate (MSG) or other natural sources of glutamate, also contributes significantly to the palatability of processed foods.

While manipulating basic tastes is essential, the magic of flavor engineering truly comes alive when aroma is integrated. It is estimated that up to 80% of what we perceive as taste is actually smell. Flavor chemists, therefore, pay special attention to volatiles - compounds that evaporate easily and contribute to the aroma of a food product. These compounds can be naturally occurring or synthetically produced to mimic natural flavors.

Texture, too, plays a critical role in our perception of food. Whether a food is crunchy, creamy, fizzy, or chewy significantly impacts how we experience it. Food manufacturers use a variety of ingredients, such as emulsifiers, stabilizers, and gelling agents, to achieve the desired mouthfeel. Even the sound that food makes when we bite into it, a concept known as 'sonic taste,' can influence our perception of its taste and freshness.

Color also influences our expectations of a food's taste and flavor. For instance, we associate yellow with a lemony flavor, red with sweetness, and green with a fresh or minty flavor. Food manufacturers use both natural and artificial colorants to make their products more visually appealing and to provide sensory cues about their likely flavors.

Apart from sensory manipulation, flavor engineers also leverage our psychological responses to food. For instance, 'vanishing caloric density' - a phenomenon where foods like puffed snacks melt quickly in our mouths - tricks our brains into thinking we're consuming fewer calories than we actually are, leading us to eat more.

The art of flavor engineering is incredibly effective, but it's also been criticized for contributing to overconsumption and, in turn, to public health issues like obesity and heart disease. As we continue to explore our relationship with processed foods, it's worth considering how we can leverage the power of flavor science to create healthier yet equally delicious food options.

Our love affair with sugar is hardwired into our biology. As the primary dietary source of readily available energy, sweetness signals that a food is high in calories and thus beneficial for survival. This evolutionary preference for sweet foods has significant implications in a world now brimming with sugar-laden processed foods.

Understanding our predilection for sugar begins with recognizing its impact on our brains. When we consume sugar, it stimulates the release of dopamine, a neurotransmitter associated with feelings of pleasure and reward. This pleasure response has been compared to the effects of addictive substances, explaining why we often crave sweet foods and find it hard to resist them.

In the context of processed foods, sugar is a dominant player. It enhances the taste of foods, makes textures more palatable, and acts as a preservative, extending the shelf life of products. It's used in everything from baked goods and cereals to sauces, dressings, and even savory snacks.

The challenge arises from the fact that our bodies were not designed to handle the large quantities of sugar now present in our diets. In prehistoric times, our ancestors would have encountered sweetness primarily in ripe fruits or honey, both consumed in moderation.

Today, with the widespread availability of sugar-sweetened foods and beverages, our consumption levels have skyrocketed.

Excessive sugar intake is associated with numerous health issues, including obesity, type 2 diabetes, heart disease, certain cancers, and dental problems. Furthermore, the metabolic effects of fructose - a component of table sugar and high-fructose corn syrup - are of particular concern. Unlike glucose, which can be used by nearly every cell in our body, fructose is primarily metabolized in the liver, where it can be turned into fat, contributing to non-alcoholic fatty liver disease and other metabolic disorders.

The food industry's use of added sugars also presents challenges in terms of consumer awareness. Food labels often list sugars under various names, like corn syrup, cane juice, maltose, or dextrose, making it difficult for consumers to recognize when sugar has been added to a product.

As we grapple with the health consequences of our sugar consumption, efforts are underway to reduce the amount of added sugar in processed foods. These strategies include reformulation, portion size reduction, and the development of alternative sweeteners. Public health interventions, such as sugar taxes, labeling initiatives, and educational campaigns, are also being implemented in various countries.

Understanding our sweet tooth and its implications is a crucial step towards making healthier dietary choices. As we continue to navigate our relationship with processed foods, it's worth exploring ways to satisfy our innate preference for sweetness in a balanced and nutritious manner.

Just as with sugar, our attraction to salt and fat is deeply rooted in our biological needs. Salt, vital for maintaining fluid balance and nerve function, is inherently appealing to our taste buds. Fat, the most energy-dense nutrient, signals a rich source of calories and contributes significantly to the mouthfeel of foods. Together, salt and fat form a powerful duo that makes processed foods highly appetizing and difficult to resist.

The allure of salt is multifaceted. Beyond its role as a basic taste, salt enhances the flavor of other ingredients, suppresses bitterness, and increases the perceived thickness of foods. It also serves important technological functions in processed foods, acting as a preservative and contributing to texture and shelf stability.

However, much like sugar, our love for salt can have health consequences. High sodium intake is associated with increased blood pressure, a major risk factor for cardiovascular diseases. Despite this, global dietary sodium intake exceeds recommended levels, driven largely by consumption of processed foods which account for the majority of our sodium intake.

Fat also plays a pivotal role in the allure of processed foods. Fats contribute to the pleasant mouthfeel of foods, delivering creaminess, smoothness, and richness that our palates enjoy. They also carry flavors, enhancing our perception of food's aroma and taste. Additionally, certain fats, particularly trans and saturated fats found in many processed foods, stimulate our brain's reward system, contributing to overeating.

Yet, dietary fats are a double-edged sword. While they are essential for nutrient absorption, cell structure, and hormone production, excessive intake, particularly of certain types of fat, can lead to obesity, heart disease, and other health problems.

To compound the issue, salt and fat are often used in tandem with sugar, creating a trifecta of tastes that hits the 'bliss point,' making processed foods hyper-palatable and promoting overconsumption.

The challenge lies in finding a balance. Salt and fat reduction strategies include food reformulation, portion control, consumer education, and public health initiatives such as nutrient profiling and food labeling. Yet, these must be achieved without sacrificing taste, a key driver of food choice. Thus, the food industry continues to explore innovative ways to reduce salt and fat in foods while maintaining their sensory appeal.

Unpacking the roles of salt and fat in our diet helps us better understand our relationship with processed foods. As we continue to seek a balance between pleasure and health in our food choices, appreciating the science behind our dietary behaviors is an important step. In the following chapters, we'll delve deeper into the implications of our processed food consumption and the potential solutions to its accompanying challenges.

W hen it comes to processed foods, the ingredients listed on the packaging often extend beyond what we traditionally think of as food. A myriad of compounds with complex names, collectively known as food additives, can be found within these products. Understanding the chemistry of these additives - their properties, roles, and potential health effects - is a fascinating yet critical aspect of navigating the world of processed foods.

Food additives are substances intentionally added to food to perform various functions. These range from improving taste, texture, and appearance, to enhancing nutritional value and increasing shelf life. The use of additives is a testament to the remarkable advances in food science and technology, enabling the production of a diverse array of processed foods.

Take preservatives, for instance. These additives prevent or slow down spoilage caused by microorganisms, thereby prolonging the shelf life of products. Sodium benzoate, commonly used in acidic foods like soft drinks, pickles, and salad dressings, inhibits the growth of bacteria, yeasts, and molds. Similarly, nitrates and nitrites, used in cured meats, are potent inhibitors of Clostridium botulinum, the bacterium responsible for botulism.

Emulsifiers, another group of additives, help mix water and oil, which naturally repel each other. In products like mayonnaise or salad dressings, emulsifiers such as lecithin maintain a stable, homogenous mixture, giving these products their smooth texture. Gelling agents, thickeners, and stabilizers, including gelatin and pectin, modify the texture of foods, contributing to their mouthfeel and overall sensory experience.

Sweeteners, both artificial and natural, replace sugar in 'sugar-free' or 'low-sugar' products. Aspartame and sucralose, popular artificial sweeteners, provide sweetness without the associated calories, making them attractive for weight management and for individuals with diabetes. However, their taste profiles and health implications have been subjects of ongoing debate.

Colorants are used to make foods visually appealing or to provide a visual cue about their flavor. Caramel coloring, derived from heated sugar, imparts a brown color to soft drinks, sauces, and confectionery. Meanwhile, beta-carotene, a naturally occurring pigment, lends a yellow-orange hue to margarine and cheese.

While these additives enhance the desirable attributes of processed foods, concerns have been raised about their potential health impacts. Some studies have linked certain food additives to health problems such as allergies, digestive issues, neurobehavioral disorders, and even cancer. However, the evidence is often mixed, and the effects are typically associated with consumption levels far above what an average person would consume.

Moreover, all food additives are subject to rigorous safety assessments by regulatory authorities such as the U.S. Food and Drug Administration (FDA) or the European Food Safety Authority (EFSA). These evaluations consider the additive's toxicity, its intake levels, and any potential health risks. Additives are only approved for use if they are deemed safe based on these assessments.

Unraveling the chemistry of food additives demystifies a significant component of processed foods. As we continue to consume these products, being informed about what we're eating and understanding the science behind it can empower us to make better dietary choices. And while the world of food additives can be complex, it's also a testament to how far we've come in our ability to preserve, enhance, and diversify our foods.

While flavor may be the star of the show when it comes to processed foods, texture plays a crucial, yet often underrated role in our food experience. It's the satisfying crunch of a potato chip, the creaminess of a pudding, the melt-in-your-mouth sensation of a high-quality chocolate. All of these sensations are meticulously crafted by an array of compounds known as texturants, which manipulate the physical properties of food to create specific mouthfeels.

Texturants, also known as texture-modifying agents, work by altering the rheology of food - the study of how substances deform and flow. In practical terms, they affect qualities like viscosity, elasticity, and gelation, essentially determining how a food behaves when it's subjected to forces, such as when it's chewed, stirred, or heated.

One group of texturants that are particularly important in processed foods are hydrocolloids, water-loving compounds that can thicken or gel liquids. These include familiar names like gelatin, pectin, and agar-agar. Each hydrocolloid has unique properties depending on its chemical structure. For instance, gelatin, derived from collagen, forms soft gels and provides a unique melt-in-the-mouth texture to foods like marshmallows and gummy bears. On the other hand, pectin, found in the cell walls of fruits, forms firm gels and is often used in making jams and jellies.

Starches are another set of vital texturants. Their ability to thicken, gel, and stabilize make them extremely versatile. For instance, in a can of soup, starch helps suspend vegetables and meat evenly, preventing them from settling at the bottom. In a cake, it contributes to the crumb structure and moistness.

Emulsifiers are texturants that mediate between water and oil, which naturally repel each other. They work by reducing the surface tension between the two, allowing them to form a stable mixture or emulsion. The result is a uniform, creamy texture, as seen in products like mayonnaise, ice cream, and chocolate. Commonly used emulsifiers include lecithin, often derived from soy or eggs, and mono- and diglycerides.

Interestingly, texturants can also impact our perception of taste. A thick, creamy yogurt may taste richer and more indulgent than a watery one, even if their flavor components are identical. The crunch of a chip can make it taste fresher, while the softness of a bread roll might make it seem less stale.

However, just like other food additives, the use of texturants is not without its controversies. Some, like carrageenan and certain modified starches, have been linked to digestive issues, while others may have potential allergenic properties. Nonetheless, texturants used in foods are evaluated for safety by regulatory bodies and are deemed safe when consumed within the approved limits.

By delving into the world of texturants, we appreciate another dimension of processed foods. The textures we experience, while often overlooked, are integral to our enjoyment of food. As our exploration of processed foods continues, we begin to grasp the immense complexity and the artistry involved in creating these everyday products.

I t is a truism to say that we eat with our eyes first. The appearance of food, its presentation, and the ambiance of the environment in which it is consumed all contribute significantly to our enjoyment of a meal. In the world of processed foods, one aspect that often dictates our first impression is the packaging.

Packaging plays a key role in the marketing of processed foods. It is the first point of contact between the consumer and the product, serving as a silent salesman that communicates brand values, product attributes, and promotional messages. With vibrant colors, attractive images, and persuasive text, packaging can significantly influence our food choices, often subconsciously.

Color, for example, can convey a multitude of messages. Red is often associated with excitement and bold flavors, and thus commonly used for snack foods and spicy products. Green, symbolizing nature and health, is frequently seen on 'natural' or 'organic' foods. Blues and purples can suggest luxury or indulgence and are commonly used in premium chocolates or desserts.

Images on the packaging can also manipulate our perceptions. Pictures of fresh fruits on a box of cereal may imply it is healthier or more natural, even if the actual fruit content is minimal. Images of happy families or children can create an association with joy and wholesomeness.

Furthermore, packaging communicates important product information, such as the ingredient list, nutrition facts, allergen statements, and health claims. However, these can be both informative and deceptive. Phrases like 'low-fat,' 'sugar-free,' or 'made with real fruit' can create a 'health halo,' causing consumers to perceive the product as healthier than it is. Similarly, serving sizes listed on the nutrition facts panel can be misleadingly small, underestimating the calories and nutrients one might actually consume.

The shape and material of the packaging can also impact our experience. Crinkly chip bags, for example, are designed to enhance the auditory experience of snacking, amplifying the perception of freshness. Glass bottles can convey a premium, artisanal feel, compared to plastic or aluminum.

However, packaging's role extends beyond marketing. It also protects the food from environmental factors, like light, air, and microbes, that can affect its quality and safety. Innovations in packaging technology have allowed for longer shelf lives, convenience, and portion control.

Understanding the psychology of food packaging enables us to make more informed choices and resist manipulative marketing tactics. As consumers, it is essential to look beyond the flashy exterior and scrutinize the contents within. As we continue to explore the world of processed foods, our journey underscores the importance of being discerning, educated consumers in the face of a complex and ever-evolving food landscape.

F ast food has become an emblem of the modern diet. Defined by its speed, convenience, and accessibility, it has seamlessly embedded itself into the fabric of contemporary life. Fast food chains dot cityscapes, suburbs, and even rural areas, their logos familiar and their offerings uniform. But what makes fast food so ubiquitous? And what implications does it have for our relationship with processed foods?

At the heart of the fast food phenomenon is its supreme convenience. In today's fast-paced society, where time is often at a premium, the speed and ease of fast food are immensely appealing. It's a meal solution that requires minimal time, effort, or culinary skills. With drive-thrus, delivery services, and mobile ordering, fast food caters to our desire for immediate gratification.

Fast food also thrives on predictability. A Big Mac in New York tastes the same as one in Tokyo, offering a familiar comfort amid the variability of life. This uniformity is achieved through the extensive use of processed foods, which can be standardized, mass-produced, and easily assembled.

These meals are meticulously engineered to be irresistibly tasty. Using a combination of high levels of sugar, salt, and fat, fast food hits the 'bliss point,' a concept we touched on in earlier chapters, stimulating our brain's reward system and encouraging repeat consumption. Moreover, the large portion sizes often provide more than one's required energy intake, contributing to overconsumption.

From a socio-economic perspective, fast food can seem economical. The immediate cost of a fast-food meal is often lower than that of fresh, whole foods, especially in food deserts where access to such foods is limited. However, the long-term costs, including the potential health implications and environmental impact, are often overlooked.

Indeed, the fast-food culture has been linked to negative health outcomes. Diets high in fast food are associated with obesity, heart disease, type 2 diabetes, and other non-communicable diseases. Moreover, while fast food menus have diversified over the years, offering salads, grilled options, and 'lite' versions, these are often overshadowed by their traditional, less healthy counterparts.

The environmental impact of the fast food industry is also significant. Issues include extensive use of single-use packaging, high levels of food waste, and resource-intensive meat and dairy products.

Despite these challenges, the allure of fast food is undeniably strong, highlighting the dominance of processed foods in our diet. As we navigate the landscape of modern eating, it is vital to be aware of these implications. By being mindful of our choices, we can enjoy the convenience of fast food while maintaining a balanced, sustainable diet. As we continue to explore the world of processed foods in the chapters to come, we'll further delve into the strategies for making healthier, more informed decisions.

When we think about processed foods, we often view them through the lens of personal health and taste preferences. However, they also play a significant role in the broader socio-economic context, influencing global food security, economic development, and social inequalities. This chapter delves into the multi-faceted socio-economic impact of processed foods.

From a food security perspective, processed foods have a crucial role to play. They can help address the challenge of feeding an ever-growing global population by improving the shelf life of food products, reducing food waste, and making nutritious food more accessible year-round. Foods like canned vegetables, fortified cereals, and preserved meats can provide essential nutrients even when fresh alternatives are unavailable or unaffordable.

Processed foods also have a major economic footprint. They drive employment and economic growth in both developed and developing countries. The food processing industry provides jobs in manufacturing, research and development, marketing, and supply chain management. The revenues generated from the sales of processed foods contribute significantly to the GDP of many nations.

However, the dominance of processed foods has also brought about social disparities. On one hand, ultra-processed foods are often cheaper and more accessible than fresh, whole foods. This is particularly true in urban food deserts, low-income areas with limited access to fresh produce. Consequently, the consumption of processed foods is often higher among lower socio-economic groups, contributing to health disparities.

On the other hand, 'healthy' processed foods, such as organic products, are often more expensive, catering to higher-income groups. The higher price point reflects the cost of organic ingredients, environmentally friendly packaging, and sustainable practices. While these products can contribute to a healthier diet, their cost can exacerbate food inequalities.

The environmental impact of processed foods also has socio-economic implications. The energy used in processing, packaging, and transporting these foods contributes to greenhouse gas emissions. The extensive use of single-use plastic packaging creates waste management issues. These environmental costs are often borne by society at large rather than the producers or consumers of these foods, an example of what economists call 'externalities.'

In conclusion, processed foods have a far-reaching socio-economic impact, touching various aspects of our lives. While they have undeniable benefits, like improving food security and driving economic growth, they also contribute to health and environmental inequalities. As we continue to navigate the world of processed foods, it's crucial to consider these broader implications and strive for a food system that is not only tasty and convenient but also equitable and sustainable.

G lobalization - the process of increasing interconnectivity and interdependence of the world's markets and businesses - has profoundly influenced the food we eat. As our planet has become a global village, foods and food practices have crossed borders, transforming diets and culinary cultures around the world. In this context, processed foods have played a central role.

The rise of multinational food corporations has been a major driver of this transformation. Companies such as Nestlé, Unilever, and PepsiCo, among others, have made their products available across the globe. A can of Coca-Cola, a pack of Oreos, or a bag of Lay's chips is recognizable and available in most corners of the world. These corporations have not only made processed foods ubiquitous but also influenced local tastes and food habits.

Globalization has facilitated the standardization of food products, which is critical for processed foods. It enables companies to maintain product consistency across different regions, ensuring that a McDonald's Big Mac or a Starbucks Frappuccino tastes the same whether you're in New York or New Delhi. This standardization is achieved through a complex global supply chain, which sources raw materials from various places, processes them in centralized factories, and distributes them worldwide.

The globalized food system has also led to the phenomenon known as 'dietary convergence'. This refers to the growing similarity of diets worldwide, characterized by increased consumption of processed foods, animal products, and sugars. Dietary convergence is linked to urbanization, rising incomes, and changing lifestyles, all facets of globalization. While this has diversified diets, it has also contributed to the global rise of obesity and non-communicable diseases, such as heart disease and diabetes.

However, the influence of globalization on food is not unidirectional. Just as Western processed foods have made their way into other parts of the world, foods from diverse culinary cultures have also been processed, packaged, and globalized. This is evident in the international popularity of foods like sushi, hummus, or tacos, which are available in ready-to-eat or easy-to-cook forms.

Moreover, the globalized food system has raised significant concerns about food sovereignty - the right of people to define their own food systems. Reliance on imported, processed foods can undermine local food cultures and make countries vulnerable to global food price fluctuations. The homogenization of diets can also lead to the loss of biodiversity, as traditional crops and local varieties are abandoned for globally traded commodities.

In conclusion, processed foods are both a product of and a driver for globalization. They have transformed and continue to reshape our food landscape, bringing about new flavors and conveniences but also new challenges. As we strive to build a sustainable, healthy, and equitable food system, it's critical to navigate these global influences with care and consideration.

There is no denying that processed foods appeal to our taste buds. With their expertly engineered combinations of salt, sugar, fat, and a host of flavorings and additives, they offer a sensory experience that can be hard to resist. Yet, this captivating dance of flavors often masks a sobering reality: many processed foods, particularly the ultra-processed varieties, fall short when it comes to nutritional quality.

Processed foods are often energy-dense, packed with calories in the form of added sugars and unhealthy fats. While these contribute to the palatability of the product, they also increase the risk of overconsumption. Given that our bodies are evolutionarily wired to crave energy-dense foods, these products can lead to a higher caloric intake than needed, contributing to weight gain and obesity.

On the other hand, many processed foods are nutrient-poor. While they deliver calories, they often lack essential vitamins, minerals, and dietary fiber. This imbalance between high energy and low nutrient content can lead to a phenomenon known as 'hidden hunger' or 'micronutrient malnutrition', where individuals may be overfed but undernourished.

Another key concern is the high amounts of salt found in many processed foods.

From canned soups and ready meals to baked goods and snacks, salt is used not just for taste but also as a preservative. High sodium intake is linked to high blood pressure, a major risk factor for heart disease and stroke.

Processed foods also tend to be low in dietary fiber, a nutrient that plays a vital role in digestive health and can help reduce the risk of chronic diseases like heart disease, type 2 diabetes, and certain types of cancer. Dietary fiber is often lost in the processing of foods, as whole grains are refined and fruits and vegetables are peeled or juiced.

Then, there's the issue of food additives, which include a range of substances like preservatives, colorants, flavor enhancers, and texturants. While these additives undergo safety assessments before they can be used in foods, concerns have been raised about their potential health impacts, particularly when consumed in large amounts over a long time. Some additives have been linked to allergies, while others are suspected to have neurotoxic or carcinogenic effects.

It's important to note that not all processed foods are equal when it comes to health. Some, like canned beans, frozen vegetables, or fortified cereals, can be part of a healthy diet. However, ultra-processed foods, characterized by extensive industrial processing and a long list of ingredients, are generally the ones associated with adverse health effects.

In the face of these challenges, the key lies in informed decision-making. Understanding the nutritional content of foods, reading labels, and making mindful choices can go a long way in balancing our love for the taste of processed foods with our need for good nutrition. As we delve further into the world of processed foods, we'll explore more strategies for maintaining this balance.

Hidden hunger, also known as micronutrient deficiency, is a form of malnutrition that occurs when intake or absorption of vitamins and minerals (also known as micronutrients) is insufficient to sustain health and development. Despite eating regular meals - and often, plenty of calories -

individuals experiencing hidden hunger lack crucial nutrients needed for their bodies to function properly. This insidious form of malnutrition is intimately linked with processed foods, which, while often energy-dense, are frequently deficient in essential nutrients.

Micronutrients, though required in small quantities, play a vital role in our health. They support a multitude of bodily functions, from energy production and immune function to blood clotting and brain development. A deficiency in any one of these micronutrients can lead to serious health problems. For example, iron deficiency can cause anemia, vitamin A deficiency can lead to blindness, and iodine deficiency can cause neurological impairments.

Processed foods, especially those that are ultra-processed, are often low in these crucial micronutrients. During processing, foods can lose many of their naturally occurring vitamins and minerals. For instance, refining grains to produce white flour, rice, or pasta can strip away the nutrient-rich germ and bran, leaving behind a product with a substantially lower nutritional value. In other cases, fruits and vegetables used in processed foods might have been harvested before peak ripeness, which means they had less time to develop a full spectrum of vitamins and minerals.

Furthermore, processed foods often substitute whole foods. A diet high in processed foods can displace healthier, nutrient-rich foods like fruits, vegetables, whole grains, and lean proteins. Therefore, even though individuals consuming a diet high in processed foods may be eating enough - or even too many - calories, they might still be deficient in essential nutrients, setting the stage for hidden hunger.

To combat this issue, some food manufacturers fortify their products with vitamins and minerals to replace those lost during processing or to boost their nutritional content. Breakfast cereals, for example, are often fortified with iron, B vitamins, and sometimes even omega-3 fatty acids. While food fortification can play a role in addressing hidden hunger, it's not a catch-all solution, as it might not provide all the necessary nutrients, and the bioavailability of added nutrients can be lower than in naturally occurring forms.

In conclusion, while processed foods provide convenience and palatability, over-reliance on them can contribute to hidden hunger. It underscores the importance of a balanced, varied diet that includes plenty of nutrient-rich whole foods. In the coming chapters, we'll explore how we can enjoy the benefits of processed foods while minimizing their potential downsides, leading us towards a healthier relationship with the foods we love.

Obesity has become a global epidemic, affecting people of all ages and socio-economic backgrounds. The World Health Organization estimates that over 650 million adults were obese in 2016, a figure that has nearly tripled since 1975. One of the key drivers of this worrying trend is the increased consumption of processed foods.

Processed foods, particularly the ultra-processed varieties, are typically high in sugars, unhealthy fats, and sodium while being low in fiber and other vital nutrients. This combination makes them energy-dense, meaning they pack a lot of calories into small volumes. They're also often designed for overconsumption, with their alluring tastes, enticing aromas, and pleasing textures.

Moreover, these foods are usually ready-to-eat or ready-to-heat, which means they require minimal preparation time, adding to their convenience factor. This has led to a shift in dietary patterns, with people increasingly relying on processed foods at the expense of healthier, home-cooked meals.

The link between processed foods and obesity can be traced to several factors. First, the high sugar and fat content of many processed foods can lead to excess calorie intake. Our bodies are evolutionarily wired to seek out sweet and fatty foods, which were scarce and valuable sources of energy in the environments in which our ancestors evolved. In today's world of abundance, this can result in overconsumption.

Second, the low fiber content of many processed foods can undermine satiety, the feeling of fullness after eating. Dietary fiber adds bulk to our diet and slows down the digestion process, helping us feel full longer. By contrast, consuming processed foods that are low in fiber can lead to increased hunger and overeating.

Third, many processed foods have a high glycemic index, which means they can rapidly spike blood sugar levels. This can result in a cycle of energy highs and lows, driving hunger and overeating.

Lastly, the omnipresence and aggressive marketing of processed foods can influence dietary behaviors, making it difficult for individuals to make healthy food choices. In many cases, the most affordable and accessible foods are the unhealthiest ones, contributing to obesity disparities among socio-economic groups.

Despite these challenges, it's important to remember that not all processed foods contribute to obesity. Some, like canned tuna, frozen vegetables, or whole grain bread, can be part of a balanced diet. Recognizing the diversity within processed foods and understanding their nutritional implications is crucial in addressing the obesity epidemic.

In the coming chapters, we will delve into strategies to navigate the world of processed foods and make healthier choices, helping to shift the scales in the fight against obesity.

s it possible to be addicted to processed foods? This question has been at the center of much scientific debate. While food addiction is not officially recognized as a clinical disorder, a growing body of evidence suggests that certain aspects of eating behavior, especially in relation to highly processed foods, share similarities with substance addiction.

Processed foods are carefully engineered to enhance their palatability. Manufacturers employ a host of techniques to intensify their products' tastes, textures, and appearances, targeting our intrinsic liking for sweet, salty, and fatty flavors. This 'hyper-palatability' can trigger a powerful response in our brains, lighting up reward pathways in a similar way to addictive substances like tobacco and alcohol.

But it's not just the taste that hooks us. Processed foods are also designed for convenience - they're easy to purchase, prepare, and consume. In our busy, fast-paced lives, the ease of popping a ready meal in the microwave or grabbing a packaged snack on-the-go is undeniably appealing. This convenience can reinforce our consumption patterns, leading us to rely increasingly on processed foods at the expense of healthier alternatives.

Moreover, processed foods are often marketed and packaged in ways that encourage overconsumption. Supersized portions, multi-packs, and 'eat-by' dates can nudge us to eat more than we need, or even want. The omnipresence of these foods - in our supermarkets, vending machines, television screens, and social media feeds - also makes them hard to resist.

The psychological concept of 'conditioned hypereating' is a useful framework to understand processed food addiction. Coined by former FDA commissioner Dr. David Kessler, it refers to a cyclical pattern of intense cravings and overconsumption triggered by cues associated with palatable foods. These cues can be external, such as the sight or smell of food, or internal, such as certain moods or thoughts. Once a person enters this cycle, it can be difficult to break free, much like in substance addiction.

However, despite these parallels, it's important to note that food and substance addictions are not identical. Unlike addictive substances, food is a basic human need. We can't simply abstain from it. Also, the concept of food addiction is complex and multifaceted, influenced by a myriad of factors including genetics, environment, psychology, and culture.

The idea of processed food addiction doesn't imply that every consumer of these foods is addicted, or that these foods are inherently 'evil'. Rather, it highlights the need for a mindful approach to our food choices. By understanding the potential addictive qualities of processed foods, we can better navigate our food environment and cultivate healthier eating habits. In the following chapters, we will discuss strategies to help achieve this balance.

C hildhood is a critical period for the development of dietary habits, preferences, and behaviors. The foods that children are exposed to, and the eating habits they develop early on, often set the stage for their dietary patterns in adulthood. Today, processed foods play a significant role in children's diets around the world, with profound implications for their health and well-being.

Processed foods are omnipresent in children's food environments, from school cafeterias to convenience stores and home pantries. These foods, which include items like sugary cereals, snack bars, hot dogs, chicken nuggets, and sodas, are often marketed directly to children, with enticing packaging, appealing tastes, and promotional tie-ins with popular cartoon characters or movies.

Children's taste preferences are significantly influenced by repeated exposure and familiarity. The more children are exposed to certain foods and flavors, the more likely they are to accept and prefer those foods. This is where processed foods, particularly those high in sugar, salt, and fat, can play a crucial role in shaping children's palates. Once children develop a liking for these hyper-palatable foods, it can be challenging to shift their preferences towards healthier alternatives.

Research has shown that high intake of processed foods in childhood is associated with a range of health issues, both immediate and long-term. These include increased risk of obesity, type 2 diabetes, and dental caries, as well as poor overall diet quality. The high sugar and sodium content of many processed foods can also lead to early development of taste preferences for sweet and salty foods, which may persist into adulthood.

Beyond the health implications, a diet dominated by processed foods can limit children's exposure to a variety of whole foods and their inherent flavors, textures, and nutritional benefits. It can also impact children's understanding and connection with food, from where it comes from to how it's prepared.

Addressing the role of processed foods in children's diets calls for a multi-pronged approach. This involves not just educating children and their caregivers about nutrition and healthy eating, but also shaping food environments to promote healthier choices. This might include improving school meal standards, regulating food marketing to children, and encouraging food manufacturers to reformulate their products to be lower in sugar, salt, and unhealthy fats.

Above all, it's about empowering children to make informed food choices. By fostering a healthy relationship with food from a young age, we can help children navigate the world of processed foods and develop eating habits that support their health and happiness, both now and in the future.

The advent of processed foods has not only altered what we eat but also how, where, and when we eat. It has significantly influenced global dietary patterns, leading to a convergence towards a 'Western' style diet characterized by high intakes of processed foods, sugars, fats, and animal-source foods, and low intakes of fruits, vegetables, and whole grains.

In the past few decades, the global food system has undergone profound changes. Technological advancements in food processing, along with globalization of food trade, have made processed foods cheaper, more diverse, and widely accessible. These foods are now available in supermarkets, convenience stores, and fast food outlets in cities and towns across the world, from metropolises to remote villages.

This global spread of processed foods has been accompanied by significant shifts in dietary patterns. Traditional diets, often rich in whole foods and locally sourced ingredients, are being replaced by diets dominated by processed foods. This dietary transition is particularly evident in rapidly urbanizing countries, where busy lifestyles, increasing incomes, and exposure to Western culture are driving a surge in consumption of processed foods.

This global dietary convergence towards a 'Western' style diet is of concern due to its implications for health and sustainability.

Diets high in processed foods are linked to increased risk of obesity, heart disease, type 2 diabetes, and certain types of cancer. At the same time, these diets are resource-intensive, contributing to environmental degradation and climate change.

However, it's important to note that not all processed foods are created equal. The category of processed foods spans a broad spectrum, from minimally processed items like canned beans and frozen vegetables to ultra-processed products like sugary drinks and instant noodles. While the latter are often high in sugars, unhealthy fats, and sodium and low in essential nutrients, the former can be part of a healthy and sustainable diet.

Navigating the global landscape of processed foods is a complex task, one that involves not just individual choices but also collective action. Policymakers, food manufacturers, retailers, and consumers all have roles to play in creating food environments that promote healthy and sustainable diets. This might involve implementing nutrition policies, reformulating food products, providing clear food labelling, and raising consumer awareness about the health and environmental impacts of different foods.

In the final chapters of this book, we will delve into the potential future of processed foods, exploring how we can leverage technology, innovation, and policy to shape this future towards one that supports both human health and planetary well-being.

As we've seen, processed foods have a significant impact on our dietary patterns and health outcomes. However, it's important to remember that the world of processed foods is not monolithic. It ranges from the most basic forms of preservation like freezing and canning, to more complex processes involved in creating ready-to-eat meals or snacks. As our understanding of nutrition and health evolves, so too does the potential to innovate within this space. There are a multitude of efforts being made towards creating healthier processed foods, harnessing technology, creativity, and science to cater to changing consumer demands.

Reformulation of existing products is one of the primary strategies being employed. This involves altering the nutritional content of processed foods to make them healthier. Reducing levels of harmful components such as salt, sugar, and trans fats, and increasing beneficial ones like fiber, whole grains, and unsaturated fats are common reformulation strategies. A great example is the move towards reducing sodium in processed meats and canned vegetables, or reducing added sugars in breakfast cereals.

Next-generation processed foods are also beginning to embrace alternative ingredients for health and sustainability reasons. Plant-based proteins, for instance, are experiencing a surge in popularity. Innovations in this area are leading to the creation of plant-based meat substitutes that mimic the taste and texture of meat, offering a potentially healthier and more sustainable alternative to traditional meat products. Other examples include the use of ancient grains in bread and pasta, or incorporating nutrient-dense vegetables and algae into snack foods.

Emerging food technologies are also promising to revolutionize the world of processed foods. Techniques like high-pressure processing, cold plasma, and pulsed light can increase the safety and shelf life of foods without the need for chemical preservatives. Similarly, precision fermentation and cellular agriculture have the potential to create animal product alternatives, like lab-grown meat or fermented proteins, which could reshape our food system in terms of both health and environmental sustainability.

Finally, there's an increasing focus on the role of the food environment in promoting healthier choices. This includes efforts to provide clearer labeling and nutrition information, to limit marketing of unhealthy foods, especially to children, and to increase the availability and affordability of healthier options.

All of these approaches recognize that processed foods are a reality of our modern food landscape, and that these foods can and should be designed to support our health and well-being. In the next chapter, we'll explore what the future might hold for processed foods, and how we can each play a part in shaping this future.

In an era where convenience often trumps all other considerations, reducing our reliance on processed foods can seem daunting. Yet, as awareness grows about the health implications associated with excessive intake of these foods, many people are seeking strategies to shift their eating habits.

Understanding the power of small, incremental changes is the first step in this journey. Rather than attempting a complete dietary overhaul, which can be overwhelming, consider making small modifications that can lead to significant improvements over time. This might involve swapping out a sugary breakfast cereal for oats topped with fresh fruit, choosing whole grain bread instead of white, or trading a bag of chips for a handful of nuts.

Incorporating more home-cooked meals into your routine is another potent strategy. Home cooking allows for complete control over the ingredients used, enabling healthier choices like reducing salt and sugar, using healthier fats, and adding more fruits, vegetables, and whole grains. This doesn't mean spending hours in the kitchen every day. Simple, nutritious meals can be prepared with minimal time and effort, and batch cooking can be a great way to have healthy meals on hand for busy days.

Mindful eating is another valuable tool in navigating our processed food environment. By slowing down and paying attention to our eating experiences, we can reconnect with our body's hunger and fullness signals, break free from automatic eating habits, and derive greater satisfaction from our meals. This can help us make more intentional food choices and reduce overconsumption, often associated with processed foods.

Understanding food labels can also go a long way in making healthier choices. By learning to decipher the information on food packages, we can make informed decisions about the processed foods we choose to include in our diets. Look for products with short ingredient lists that contain recognizable items, with minimal added sugars, sodium, and unhealthy fats.

Cultivating a supportive social environment can be a powerful enabler of dietary change. This might involve seeking support from family and friends, joining a community with shared health goals, or even advocating for healthier food environments in schools, workplaces, and local communities.

Lastly, remember to exercise self-compassion and patience. Changing dietary habits is a process that takes time and will inevitably involve some setbacks. Each meal is a new opportunity to make healthier choices, and every small change counts.

In our final chapter, we will delve into the potential future of processed foods, exploring how we can leverage the power of innovation and policy to shape a food landscape that supports both human health and planetary well-being.

The food landscape of the future will undoubtedly include processed foods. They are woven into the fabric of our society, providing convenience, affordability, and variety in our diets. But the nature of these foods, their health impact, and their role in our diets can, and likely will, change.

As we have seen, efforts are already underway to transform the processed food landscape. From reformulating existing products to reduce harmful ingredients to leveraging emerging technologies to create next-generation foods, the face of processed foods is evolving. The rise of plant-based proteins, lab-grown meat, and nutrient-fortified foods point to a future where processed foods could be designed to deliver both taste and health.

Consumer demand will play a crucial role in shaping this future. As awareness grows about the health and environmental implications of our food choices, consumers are increasingly seeking out healthier, more sustainable options. This demand can drive innovation in the food industry, encouraging the development of products that meet these evolving preferences.

Policy and regulation will also be instrumental in shaping the future of processed foods. Nutrition policies can incentivize food manufacturers to reformulate their products, while regulations on food marketing, labeling, and taxes can influence consumer behavior. School food programs and workplace wellness initiatives can also play a role in promoting healthier food environments.

While technology and innovation hold promise for creating healthier processed foods, the importance of whole foods should not be underestimated. Fruits, vegetables, whole grains, legumes, nuts, and seeds offer a symphony of nutrients in their natural form, and eating these foods in variety and abundance will continue to be the cornerstone of a healthy diet.

In a world where processed foods are here to stay, the challenge lies in striking the right balance. Balancing the convenience and enjoyment of processed foods with the health benefits of whole foods. Balancing individual responsibility with the role of policy and industry in shaping our food environments. Balancing the need for global dietary convergence with respect for cultural diversity and traditional diets.

The future of food is not a one-size-fits-all proposition, but rather a rich tapestry of possibilities that reflect our diverse needs, values, and aspirations. As we look towards this future, let's remember that we are all stakeholders in our food system, and we each have a role to play in shaping a food landscape that nourishes both people and planet.

In closing, "The Processed Pantry: Our Love Affair with Engineered Eats" invites you, the reader, to think critically about your relationship with processed foods and to explore new ways of engaging with our food system. May this journey of discovery inspire you to savor the pleasures of eating, to cherish the power of food to nourish and heal, and to join the collective effort to create a healthier, more sustainable food future.